UPDATED

Pregnancy
and
Fibromyalgia

Melissa Reynolds

Also by
Melissa Reynolds

Melissa vs Fibromyalgia:
My Journey Fighting Chronic Pain, Chronic Fatigue and Insomnia

Fibromyalgia Framework (workbook)

Praise for Melissa and Her Books

"Oh I loved it [*Pregnancy and Fibromyalgia*] so much! I don't think I would have coped through my pregnancy without it."

—A Fibro Mama

"Lived experience + self-awareness + systems thinking + good storytelling is golden. Add brevity and it's priceless. Melissa's book is priceless."

—Danny van Leeuwen, Opa, RN, MPH, CPHQ
Health Hats (www.health-hats.com)

"Pregnancy and Fibromyalgia is a short, easy-to-digest run-down of things you can expect during a fibro pregnancy, and how to navigate them."

—Diane Murray
Spoonie Living (blog.spoonieliving.com)

"An invaluable resource for fibro baby mammas."

—Caz
Invisibly Me (www.invisiblyme.com)

"Melissa is a brilliant writer and I enjoy her work. I recommend her book if you have fibromyalgia or know someone who does."

—Jessie

"Melissa provides numerous tips on how to effectively manage fibromyalgia while pregnant and why these steps are important. She gives insight to her pregnancies and how she coped with each one."

—B Clevinger

*Thank you to those few people I have met
who have truly attempted to understand
this beast I fight.*

Contents

UPDATED EDITION

Pregnancy
and
Fibromyalgia

Melissa Reynolds

Disclaimer

None of the content specified in this book is to be treated as medical advice and not as a replacement for a professional healthcare physician. I am not an expert in Fibromyalgia, Chronic Fatigue Syndrome or Myofascial Pain Syndrome – I am an expert in my experience. I share my experiences and research to help you be your own advocate and to make the experience of this illness more visible.

You will note the expectation that you will do your own research. I provide the information so that you can read it and discuss it with your doctor. This enables you to make informed choices and be part of the decisions that affect you and your baby.

Congratulations! You're a Fibro Parent (or Want to Be)

If you've had Fibromyalgia (or any similar chronic illness) for any amount of time, you likely already know that there is no magic pill. No one else can do the work for you. You have probably built a crap-load of resilience; you know yourself and your boundaries (I know, I'm still working on this); and you work hard to be well every day. Additionally, you can't take a day off.

However, the good news is that this will help you with pregnancy.

It's a marathon, but it's a struggle with an end date.

I can give you tips for what worked for me, you can read about Fibromyalgia and pregnancy, and you can read (the practically non-existent but slowly multiplying information) about pregnancy with Fibromyalgia, but in the end, it is you putting one foot in front of the other.

That's how we live, right?

It is my hope that this book will help you to get through your pregnancy or help you to see that a family can be achievable with Fibromyalgia. I gather research, my experience and anecdotal experience together in key areas in this book: pregnancy, nursing and having tiny children.

It isn't as simple as doing everything I did; human beings are complex, and Fibromyalgia magnifies this complexity. Where I found pregnancy made my symptoms worse, others have found it gave them a symptom holiday. Where I found nursing a major energy drain, others managed to feed happily for over 12 months.

Whatever place on the spectrum you are on, it is my hope that something here will help you on your journey. I hope you get to enjoy the miraculous event that making a baby is.

Because it truly is spectacular.

Fibromyalgia and Pregnancy: The Literature

There is a disappointing lack of literature on pregnancy and Fibromyalgia. Doctors can't seem to decide if pregnancy makes Fibromyalgia symptoms worse or better. I have met a pain specialist who says that pregnancy doesn't impact Fibromyalgia or vice versa.

I beg to differ.

Your body is a whole entity. What affects one part has an impact on the rest. For example, worsening sleep due to back pain, which is triggered, in part, by fibro and pregnancy, causes more pain and more fatigue.

Pregnancy is a big energy drainer; those with Fibromyalgia just don't have much to begin with. I've provided a few pertinent articles below and summarised the key learning from my reading.

Here's a few key articles I've found:

1. A study entitled *The Effect of Reproductive Events and Alterations of Sex Hormone Levels on the Symptoms of Fibromyalgia* (1997) found that most of the women studied found the third trimester worsened their symptoms, that the Fibromyalgia had no

adverse effect on the outcome of the pregnancy or the baby's health, and the premenstrual symptoms were reported worse in 72% of patients.

2. Jacob Teitelbaum, MD, Medical Director of the Fibromyalgia and Fatigue Centers and author of important Fibromyalgia treatment book *From Fatigued to Fantastic!* (2007), wrote an article about pregnancy with Fibromyalgia, *Pregnancy in Chronic Fatigue Syndrome and Fibromyalgia*, on The Environmental Illness Resource. In it, he recommends supplements to support pregnancy and medicines to avoid. Generally, I love Dr T., but his assumption that most women experience an improvement of symptoms during pregnancy was very wrong for me. He also states that he doesn't believe breastfeeding to be too tiring, but I found it to be very energy draining.

3. The article *Fibromyalgia and Pregnancy: Expert Q&A* on Healthline discusses pregnancy and Fibromyalgia, acknowledging the difficulty that arises for women with Fibromyalgia, particularly until the baby sleeps better.

4. Webmd's article *Fibromyalgia and Pregnancy* (2016) highlights the lack of studies on women with Fibromyalgia during pregnancy and the increase in pain: *"There are few studies on fibromyalgia in pregnant women. However, a study at Temple University found that women with fibromyalgia had more symptoms of pain during pregnancy than women who did not have fibromyalgia. Also, fibromyalgia symptoms seemed to be exacerbated during pregnancy."* This is certainly my finding, but I have heard of

those who found pregnancy to be like a holiday from their symptoms.

5. The National Fibromyalgia and Chronic Pain Association provides seven tips for coping with Fibromyalgia during pregnancy, including educate yourself and family and friends, manage pain, get some help and have no expectations.

Here are the key things you need to know:

1. Try to have the Fibromyalgia managed well prior to falling pregnant. This made a huge difference for me with my third pregnancy.

2. You may experience a betterment or a worsening of your symptoms. In my survey, it was nearly 50/50. But it is more likely that you will experience a flare up after pregnancy, 68.4% of respondents reported a severe flare up after the birth of their baby.

3. Managing Fibromyalgia, with or without pregnancy, is a matter of self-care and healthy choices: eat well; exercise as best you can; avoid stress; rest; sleep.

4. Create a pain management plan. This is a loaded topic. Prior to my first pregnancy, I wasn't managing my pain well. So, during my pregnancy, due to the lack of information and appropriately educated medical professionals, I remained under-treated – until I was given codeine in my second trimester (really, nothing to codeine!).

Do your research and discuss the costs and benefits with an appropriately educated health professional, someone who understands that untreated pain has health risks to both mother and baby. Through my research, I have found that under-treated pain can have negative health consequences. The article *Amitriptyline* (2014) from the Best Use of Medicine in Pregnancy (BUMPS) website puts it this way when considering continuing amitriptyline, or any medication during pregnancy: *"Remaining well is particularly important during pregnancy and while caring for a baby. For some women treatment with amitriptyline in pregnancy may be necessary."*

5. Plan for the first months. Most of the literature identifies the need for support, especially post-birth and for the first six months when the Fibromyalgia is likely to be flared due to the sleep deprivation and being off medications for breastfeeding.

Conclusion

There is no reason that a woman with Fibromyalgia should avoid having children. With planning, understanding and a heavy dose of acceptance of whatever happens, happens, it can be managed. My aim is to share my learning and experience so that others are not grappling in the dark as I was.

Fertility and Fibromyalgia: Not an Area of Concern, According to the Research

"There is scant evidence that fibromyalgia may interfere with a woman's chance to get pregnant."

Dr. Ananya Mandal, MD
Fibromyalgia Fertility/Pregnancy (2013)

Despite the symptoms of Fibromyalgia usually affecting menstruation and pregnancy symptoms, it does not appear to effect fertility.

There is an article entitled *Treating Infertility in Fibromyalgia – An Information Sheet for Couples* (2017) written by Jacob Teitelbaum, MD, on the ProHealth website that doesn't explain whether Fibromyalgia affects fertility and doesn't really talk about infertility beyond the statistic that it affects 1 in 6 couples and can be more common in Fibromyalgia due to hypothyroidism, nutritional deficiencies or PCOS. The article does go on to give both the intending to be pregnant parent and the inseminating parent tips for increasing fertility.

Tips include a broad spectrum multivitamin, thyroid support, avoiding certain things that can impede fertility, optimise iron levels and watch the level of folic acid. There is also a list of supplements for the inseminating parent.

As the author of the previous article alludes to, fertility issues may be more likely caused by illnesses that are correlated with Fibromyalgia as opposed to being caused by Fibromyalgia itself. Endometriosis is one such illness that is associated with Fibromyalgia and infertility.

The article *Fibromyalgia and Fertility* (2017) by Tiffany Vance-Huffman on the Fibromyalgia Treating website also discusses this "inadvertent" link.

Conclusion

The research suggests that it is not the Fibromyalgia per say that affects fertility, but other issues that can be comorbid with Fibromyalgia.

Lots of Natural Pain Relief Suggestions

Pain was a big issue for me during and after pregnancy. At least after labour, a lot more medicines are considered safe. Before I dive into the chapter on pain relief and my experience of pregnancy with Fibromyalgia, I include this list which contains suitable options for before, during and after pregnancy.

The List:

- Stay hydrated
- Nourish yourself with the best food you can manage (put down the white carbs! Unless that's the only thing your tummy can take today)
- Heat pack
- Warm bath (add Epsom salts)
- Warm shower
- Stretch
- Pelvic tilts/cat and cow pose
- Gentle walking
- Rest
- Pace - alternate activity with rest

- Meditation, especially pain relief focused. Look up *Guided Mindfulness Meditation on Coping with Pain (20 Minutes) (2016)* on YouTube.
- Avoid things that cause pain
- Trigger point cane massager
- Self-massage
- Massage from a partner
- Massage by a massage therapist
- Osteopathy
- Chiropractic
- Ice pack
- Restorative yoga poses (like child's pose)
- Non-medicinal pain cream (like Deep Heat)
- Magnesium oil (especially on your calves at bedtime to avoid waking with cramps)
- Essential oils that are safe for pregnancy (see note below)
- Chamomile tea
- Peppermint tea (for tummy upsets)
- Go to bed early
- For a severe headache: feet in hot water, ice pack around neck
- For headaches or muscle tension: Peppermint oil with a carrier oil (I always have coconut oil on hand and it's less greasy than others) on the temples (see note below).
- Check all nutrient levels and supplement where needed – especially magnesium and iron.

- Lavender oil massaged into your feet or neck/temples if you can handle the smell (see note below).
- Homeopathic remedies (check with an experienced practitioner)
- Physiotherapy with acupuncture – especially for trigger points. When pregnant ensure the practitioner understands there are points to avoid during pregnancy.
- Go for a swim or walk in a heated pool
- Use a pregnancy pillow (comfort in bed is key)
- Go to a prenatal yoga class

I haven't personally tried the below options but they are advertised for pregnant women and appear to have some good health benefits (please research!):

- Elsmore Oil
- Bio-Strath Elixir
- 5-W for the final stages of pregnancy and childbirth
- Artemis Pregnancy Tea – In addition to the belief that raspberry leaf can aid in shortening labour, the ingredients in this tea are packed with nutrients.
- Flax Bloom
- Blackthorn Elixir
- Rebozo Technique - basically using a long piece of cloth to support the stomach and back and also for gentle movement during the third trimester and delivery.

A note about essential oils:

Please note that it is not recommended to ingest oils during pregnancy (I'd question ingesting them at all, but you will research and decide for yourself) or to use essential oils during the first trimester. For the same reasons we try to minimise medicine use in pregnancy, there isn't enough data to consider it safe.

This article is a good starting point for your research: *Using Essential Oils Safely for Pregnant or Nursing Mamas* (2015) on The Hippy Homemaker.

Pain Management in Pregnancy with Fibromyalgia

There is an issue that gets me fired up, but it's difficult to make recommendations in this area due to the complexity of it: pain relief in pregnancy.

It makes me so sad when I hear of people being ignored and left in tremendous levels of pain due to too conservative doctors. I heard of one woman recently who was basically harassed about medicinal choices in pregnancy and had two doctors who disagreed about the use of a medicine.

It's also an area that made a difference between my first and second pregnancies. Pain relief was the difference between misery and coping. This is in general life with chronic pain and in pregnancy, only in pregnancy, you have less options.

There are resources available that can help you make the decision of what to stay on and what to go off. Your body is a whole: what affects one system will have an effect on another.

A ton of anecdotal evidence exists for many medicines. There was a category system for rating the safety of medicines in pregnancy, which was updated in 2015 and now revolves around a system of gathering information and making an informed decision with costs and benefits in mind (*FDA Pregnancy Risk Information: An Update* on *Drugs.com*). It does make the decision making for a very tired, sore pregnant person a bit more difficult, because you have to read through a heap of scary sounding information, so I often fall back to the old category rating as a guide.

There are some medicines that are categorically unsafe for pregnancy. There are a lot of medicines that they just don't know enough about, performing experiments on pregnant people, particularly involving something that may harm a baby, would be unethical. So literature relies on data provided by pregnant people. The website *Mother to Baby* provides fact sheets, access to professionals to speak to about medicine in pregnancy and more. I also always check *drugs.com* when I am considering a medicine.

Let me tell you that your quality of life counts. It counts during these 40 or so weeks of pregnancy and it matters during nursing and parenting. It also matters if children aren't a factor in your life.

If you feel your doctor is being too conservative, please seek a second opinion. Ultimately, you will need to take costs and benefits into account. It will also be you going through each day through pregnancy and labour and parenting.

Your opinion counts.

You do not have to be miserable, there's also research that suggests that undertreated pain can negatively affect the pregnancy (Malaika Babb et al, *Treating pain during pregnancy* from ncbi.nlm.gov).

As an example, amitriptyline is a category C medicine by the old category system. There's animal research that suggests it's unsafe (in very high doses, far higher than one would take). There's also anecdotal human evidence that it's potentially safe. I cannot sleep without it and I sleep very poorly in pregnancy due to pain and pregnancy induced "super" insomnia. I could not have coped going off it. My doctor, a specialist and I agreed that in my context the benefits outweighed potential risks – and we made this cost versus benefit analysis for each pregnancy.

So, after trying all of the natural pain relief mechanisms, if you're still in severe pain, what can you do?

Advanced Pain Relief in Pregnancy

I can only share what worked for me. You need to do your research, especially around medicines in pregnancy. Chat everything through with your doctor. If you feel that your doctor is being too conservative and you are struggling, find another doctor to speak with.

Please note I am providing information for you to make your own choices I don't mind if you prefer no medicines at all or take several; that's between you and your doctor/medical team.

- Check the *www.drugs.com* site for information about pregnancy and breastfeeding with the medicines you are on.
- Check *www.mothertobaby.org* for the fact sheets.
- This article also lists several key medicines by name so it is worth a read: "*Severe or chronic pain, if left untreated or inadequately*

treated, can have adverse effects on both the mother and the fetus" (*Non-Obstetric Pain in Pregnancy,* 2008, Dr Abdul Lalkhen & Dr Kate Grady; check references).

- *"Topical NSAIDs [gels] generally result in negligible blood levels and would be considered to be relatively safe in pregnancy although absorption is increased by use over a large surface area or the application of heat"* (from *Analgesics and Pain Relief in Pregnancy and Breastfeeding,* 2011, Michael McCullough; check references).

Continuing the theme:

- This doctor suggests NSAIDS are safe in the second trimester, absolutely contraindicated after week 32 (*Rheumatoid, Psoriatic Arthritis & Pregnancy: All Queries Answered,* 2018, Dr Nilesh Nolkha; check references).
- Excellent article exploring pain, pregnancy and chronic illness (*Pain, Pregnancy & Prescriptions: Why You Should Treat Your Pain and How to Manage Safely (While Trying To Conceive & Pregnant),* 2018, Katarina Zulak; check references).
- *Low Dose Naltrexone in Pregnancy* (n.d.) presentation by Dr Phil Boyle (check references)
- *Interview with Dr. Phil Boyle,* Director of the NaPro Fertility Care Clinic in Dublin, Ireland (check references).

Low Dose Naltrexone and Pregnancy – An Area to Research Carefully

I began reading about low dose naltrexone (LDN) while I was pregnant with my second baby. After devouring all of the positive research, I decided to start taking it after I finished nursing him.

I learned afterward that it is *potentially* safe to take LDN until the 37th week of pregnancy and for breastfeeding. I believe this is to be because you generally go into labour anytime from 37-42 weeks and you may need opioids during the labour – I did for all of my labours.

There are fertility clinics that use LDN specifically to help women with autoimmune conditions to maintain a pregnancy. So there are a lot of women who have been given it for pregnancy. But this is a decision you and your doctor must make after looking at the available evidence, which includes anecdotal evidence as research into medicines during pregnancy would be unethical.

There are no long-term studies as of yet. As with all medicine use in pregnancy, it would be a matter of balancing cost versus benefits. Would the LDN help more than the potential risks?

Dr Phil Boyle presents his findings in a presentation – *Low Dose Naltrexone in Pregnancy* (n.d.), showing the comparison of outcomes between those in his clinic that used LDN and those that didn't, and the results were fairly positive. On the flipside of that, a study on animals using LDN during pregnancy was not-so positive, as documented on the LDN Now website.

It is considered potentially safe for breastfeeding – this is discussed on Drugs.com discusses this in the article *Naltrexone Use While Breasting* (n.d.): *"Limited data indicate that naltrexone is minimally excreted into breast milk. If naltrexone is required by the mother, it is not a reason to discontinue breastfeeding."*

Please note: This is a finding on the usual dose of Naltrexone, often used to help detox off drugs.

Over a period of 18 months LDN had helped me so much that when I became pregnant with my third son, my doctor and I decided that there were more than enough benefits and not enough risks to be worried. I had a much better pregnancy, even with severe pelvis issues that saw me put off work in the second trimester and using crutches.

I stayed on LDN until week 37, had my baby at 38 weeks and 3 days and resumed LDN five days postpartum. For me this was the right choice and made a huge difference to my quality of life.

Pregnancy with Fibromyalgia: Tools for Managing Early Pregnancy Symptoms

For a person with Fibromyalgia, motherhood is not a short sprint. It's an epic marathon spanning pregnancy, labour and baby's first year. So it's really important to get your pregnancy wellness plan underway fast. Here are some things I have learnt for tackling the early pregnancy symptoms:

Sleep

I tried as best as I could, but sleep in normal life is difficult for me, in pregnancy it is even trickier. I had a maternity pillow and a pillow for between my legs. I utilised body scan meditations to encourage certain parts of my body to relax.

I found that the chronic fatigue was greatly flared up and the amount of sleep I got was almost directly related to my nausea levels.

Pacing

The work/rest cycle is really best for managing pain, fatigue and pregnancy. Sometimes it may feel as if the rest needs to be longer than the work portion, but try to allow that as best you can. If you are working or managing children, try to take at least one rest per day – even if it is a 10 minute meditation in the car at the side of the road (I did this before I picked my kids up from their carer's house). Try to ensure you get a few decent rests on the weekend.

Meditation

As a stubborn (my body, not me!) non-napper and a troubled sleeper, meditation is a lifesaver. It is useful first thing if you wake too early and cannot get back to sleep. It can be used midday, whenever you need a lie down – or it can be used right before bed. You can choose simple breath-focused meditation; you can listen to guided meditation or you can do body scans. You can choose meditations specifically for pain or pregnancy. There's a heap available on YouTube to try. I like this video: *Pregnancy Relaxation – Guided Meditation for Pregnant Women* on YouTube. I've written an extended my post about meditation and Fibromyalgia on my blog called "Giant Meditation Post."

Exercise

Walking is a big part of my usual pain management plan, and this is no different in pregnancy. During my first pregnancy, I was able to continue gentle 20-30 minute walks all around our neighbourhood after the hardest weeks were over. During the worst weeks, I managed about 10 minutes a day. Yoga was off the menu for me for all three pregnancies due to post-exertion malaise and pelvis issues. Your body will tell you. Anything you did before is usually okay during pregnancy.

Search up *Top Three Yoga Poses for Pregnancy* by Sarah Beth Yoga on YouTube. And this article *5 Exercises to Help Get Rid of Back Pain During Pregnancy.*

Fuel

I needed smaller amounts of food more often, so I adjusted my meals to suit this and this helped stabilise my energy levels and avoid the more severe nausea. When I was the sickest and unable to eat, I found that gently coaxing my tummy back to food – diluted orange juice, small amounts of milk, toast and then whatever I fancied – worked. Crackers by the bed for midnight or 3am snacks were a handy hack! So was a little yogurt right before bed; the protein helped to carry me through. I also took the Energy Revitalisation Formula (a powdered multivitamin) to help my general nutritional needs.

Pain Management Plan

My doctor helped me to put together a system for dealing with the pain using as minimal medicinal input as possible. My big struggle has always been my neck, during my first two pregnancies, I needed paracetamol and codeine in order to get any sleep. You may like to look into homeopathic remedies, using an experienced practitioner's advice. My doctor is a big fan, and I used Crampmed by Naturo Pharm. I always utilise my natural pain relief mechanisms as listed earlier.

Nausea

This is pretty much unavoidable, but I have a few tricks for reducing it:

- Keep your tummy from getting empty
- Don't get too fatigued (using the tools above)
- Ginger lozenges or mints
- A couple of drops of peppermint essential oil topically (this was a very personal choice given they don't have research on the use of essential oils in early pregnancy)
- Acupuncture for nausea in the wrist point or the seasickness bands that hold pressure in the same point.

Going to the Bathroom ALL the Time

I can't really help with this; I did avoid anything other than water after 3pm, but otherwise, just go with the flow!

Plan

If you're at all like me, you will find comfort in planning ahead. And write everything down because it may fall out of your head. Figure out potential parental leave options early.

Enjoy

You're growing a tiny human! Revel in that a little. Also enjoy the things you can do now and will have to give up later (Weird Fact: I did certain stretches and legs on a chair pose like crazy because I knew I'd have to give them up from week 16 or so!)

Weeks 7-10

"Week seven was when things started to turn around a little. I had been rather sick in week six and managed to claw my way back by eating every two or three hours, going to bed early and limiting activity."

Fibro Mama Pregnancy Diaries (Take Two)

Pregnancy with Fibromyalgia: Second Trimester

The second trimester is meant to be the "magical" trimester. I certainly never found anything magical about pregnancy, but the second and third times around, I truly found a distinction between the first and second trimesters: a real diminishing of symptoms. The nausea vanished, the more extreme fatigue receded and my low back pain eased. For a time.

I had my coping mechanisms well in place. I already had a plan for coping with the third trimester, labour and the first weeks.

Sleep, of course, was difficult as my neck and shoulders hate (with a capital H) lying on my sides. Every time I changed positions, which was often, I woke. But meditation around lunch time for 20 or 30 minutes really helped me to cope.

Here's what I did to be well:

- Energy Revitalisation Formula a general multivitamin to support nutrition for those with Fibromyalgia, any pregnancy multi is a good idea.
- Making better food choices – once I wasn't so sick.

- Exercise as I could – this meant walking as I could, being generally active (using 8000+ steps a day until the pelvis pain incapacitated me in the third pregnancy) and some gentle resistance work (superman, pelvic tilts and lots of pelvic floors).
- Stretch – often!
- Heat pack – not only does it ease pain, but I had to sit or lie down with it for it to stay on my neck or back.
- Sleep and rest – bed at a good time, meditation about lunchtime.
- Journaling – taking time to write "mama notes" documenting the pre-schooler, the toddler and the pregnancy.
- Physio – every 2 weeks.

Conclusion

As the trimester progressed and sleep deteriorated (due to worsening back and pelvis pain), it did become more of a slog. However, a heavy dose of acceptance helped – pregnancy is a trying time for anybody, it is finite and I do all I can to help myself.

For my third pregnancy, it also helped to be able to say things like, "These are my last first kicks," "This is the last time I will have to cope with pregnancy-caused backache" and "This is my last second trimester"!

Weeks 15-17

"The absence of stress and too many work hours really helped me cope physically. Although the burden on my husband is not light."

Fibro Mama Pregnancy Diaries (Take Two)

Pregnancy with Fibromyalgia: The Third Trimester

It is no secret that the third trimester of pregnancy is a trying time. Especially if you have Fibromyalgia and any of the comorbid disorders that can go hand-in-hand with it.

I struggled so much with my first pregnancy that I was very scared of the prospect of a second. However, I muddled through the second and third pregnancies with the following aids:

Acupuncture

This helped with nausea in the first trimester and then with the pain as the pregnancy progressed. In the third trimester I visited my physiotherapist (who performs acupuncture) regularly.

Keep moving

I walked until the last day of my pregnancy with my first. With my second I did what I could. With my second I was pretty much house-bound for the final weeks of the pregnancy but the entire time I continued to move as much as I could. I stretched when I couldn't walk.

Sleep

Find what will help. I had a great full body pillow that I curled around. Sleep was still difficult, but it helped.

Rest

Don't stand when you can sit or sit when you can lie down! Don't become a couch blob, but take it easy! Meditate.

Eat Healthily

I fell in love with semolina porridge (or sooji, as my Indian in-laws know it), it became my power dish. Try to really think of food as fuel. Fruit, vegetables, whole grains, protein. This may be a good area to get some advice in as I have certainly found that nutrition has a big impact on health.

Write a Journal

Try to focus on the beautiful baby you will be given and that will help you to remember that this time will pass!

Stop Work as Soon as You Can

If it becomes a real struggle and you are so sore that you can't sit down, like I was, then try to give it up as soon as possible.

A quick note on positioning

Don't spend your third trimester laying back and making your back seem like a hammock. Spend time on all fours and sit up straight so baby will use your belly as a hammock. You'll want to avoid back to back positioning. Back labour is mean.

There are a lot of options for belly support belts, from below the belly only to full top and bottom belly belts. I found the top and bottom far too restrictive, therefore didn't use it enough. There are some great under belly options available if you care to Google.

A note on pelvis and low back pain:

If your pain in the low back feels severe, if your pelvis feels sore or unstable then you may have symphysis pubis disorder. This is no joke. I was fobbed off with the "fibro" basket and suffered for it. There's a lot you can do. Support that belly.

Conclusion

One thing you definitely need to do is check your iron levels. Ask the doctor, when your results come in, what the level is (it's a large range), and if it's low already, ask for an easily digestible supplement. It's standard here to wait until week 28 before testing, and by then, I had become so low that my stores were wiped, making life much harder than it needed to be. I was beside myself exhausted. And for good reason. Finally, know that there is a finite time that you are pregnant for. Try to enjoy it! Stockpile the rest!

Weeks 36-38

"Unfortunately, we found that my iron levels had completely depleted and I had to quickly have an iron injection in week 37. It certainly explained why I had been so exhausted, lethargic, nauseas and in so much pain. Within days of the injection, I felt so much better. It was amazing. I hadn't realised how sick I had gotten."

Fibro Mama Pregnancy Diaries (Take Two)

Labour with Fibromyalgia

Labour is a unique event for every woman, every time she encounters it. Research suggests that Fibromyalgia doesn't affect labour, except that those with Fibromyalgia may tire more easily and feel more pain.

I have had three very different experiences. My first was posterior (back to back), which caused severe back pain for the entirety of the 20 hour ordeal. My second had the cord wrapped around him three times, which is unusual. I also had undiagnosed symphysis pubis disorder, which definitely made pushing torturous. With my third, I experienced two days of pre-labour, period-like pains, a day and a night of early labour and then just three hours of active labour. I pushed him out in 24 minutes!

In my eCourse *Fibro Mama Pregnancy and Fibromyalgia*, I give lots of tips for coping in early labour as well as guide participants through making their own plan for the third trimester, early labour and the first six weeks.

Your midwife/lead maternity carer/obstetrician should go over this with you. Nothing I suggest supersedes their ideas. But there are a few things that could help in the last weeks and those early hours of labour.

- Heat pack - this was divine on my back in early labour all times.

- Warm bath/shower
- Cat/cow pose - I did a lot of these throughout all of my pregnancies and labour; I think it's instinctual to get on all fours and relieve your back in this way.
- Pelvic rocking - I spent a lot of time on my Swiss ball doing this.
- Meditation - I did this one a lot. You can type in "labour visualisation meditation" into YouTube and lots of results come up.
- Rest - it is good to stay active but balance it with rest. I was charging around when labour began with my second, I ended up tired and still pregnant!
- A good movie - choose a movie or TV show that can keep you occupied for the time.
- A gentle walk
- Keep hydrated and keep eating light, gentle foods for as long as possible as it could be a while from early labour to eating after baby.
- Prepare your support person to advocate for you when you are unable to do so yourself.

The Delivery

"While it was a long, hard, painful labour, I can clearly recall the care of the many professionals I encountered, my midwife being the lead. I felt looked after and that my baby was being carefully monitored. The after care, during which I haemorrhaged, was also spectacular. This is what I remember the most from my experience. And it was dramatically different from my first labour, for this I'm grateful."

Fibro Mama Pregnancy Diaries (Take Two)

A Letter to Midwives

I remember it vividly. Sitting in a low, grey chair, behind a curtain with a double breast pump at work, tears streaming down my face. I started crying that morning and couldn't stop. It was three days after a hard pregnancy and delivery, and I'd had very little sleep. The midwife said my Fibromyalgia must be pretty bad. I didn't say anything at the time, but I can't stop thinking about it.

I want to tell her that it's not.

I usually cope very well. But she saw me on one of the worst days of my life. After a pregnancy of increasing pain and decreasing sleep. After a hard labour. After three days of very little sleep, with a baby who couldn't get enough food from me. Hideous pain in my breasts and in my stitches. To top it off, my husband wasn't allowed to stay. So I was alone with this baby from 9pm to 9am.

The midwives on the nightshift didn't help very much. They latched baby on and left. They didn't see the pain caused by his latch becoming shallower as he drank. If I took him off to try to re latch, he'd refuse it.

On that last day, the best things happened. And only because I couldn't stop crying. They taught me to express milk for my baby to drink via the bottle. This meant I was able to see that my baby had enough food, that I could bother my very sore breasts only three-hourly and that I had an element of control.

This enabled me to give my baby breast milk exclusively for eight weeks, instead of just that first week.

We need options. I was committed to feeding my baby, but I needed the option to help me do that. I am so thankful for this, so thankful that they were not judgemental. 'Cause, damn, breastfeeding hurt me!

They also let my husband stay on the final night.

He is why I managed. We took turns feeding, so I got some sleep. I also had a person to experience it all with me. Alone, in pain, with a screaming baby is not a key for coping.

What I want to tell all midwives is that my experience of Fibromyalgia isn't so bad - there are people who have it worse.

Please educate yourselves so that you can help. Even if you know enough to know that the husband or a support person needs to stay to help.

A person with Fibromyalgia is likely to have a higher perception of the pain.

They are more likely to have had a very painful pregnancy.

They are more prone to emotional changes – when you're in a lot of pain and so tired you can't think straight; you can't keep your emotions on an even keel.

So please know this. Please be aware. We need a little extra help.

Nursing with Fibromyalgia

L ike many areas of living with Fibromyalgia, I have found there to be little information on nursing with Fibromyalgia. There are a few articles, like the one on Fibromyalgia Symptoms that mentions research but provides no links: "Numerous studies have been done evaluating how fibromyalgia influences breastfeeding. These studies all indicate that it is very hard to breastfeed with fibromyalgia."

The Fibromyalgia Health Center on WebMD posted an article in 2004 referencing a new study about nursing with Fibromyalgia. This study was very small, with just nine mothers included:

"All nine women felt that they were not successful in their attempts to breastfeed, and felt frustrated," Schaefer writes. Difficulties included muscle soreness, pain, and stiffness; fatigue; a perceived shortage of breast milk; and sore nipples."

The article lists a few tips from the study which includes good nutrition, proper rest and paying attention to where and how you are nursing.

In a 2017 survey I collected to inform my writing, I received surprising results for the question around nursing. According to it, 15% didn't manage to nurse, 5.3% exclusively expressed, 21.1% nursed for six months and 12 months each; and a whopping 38.8% managed to nurse for more than 12 months. (Go you!)

Again, this is a small sample size and it is not scientifically constructed – I accepted all responses and didn't screen anyone out. It is a useful counterpoint to the research above.

Having had three children now, I can confirm that every experience is different. As with all areas of this illness, my experience may not be the same as another's, so my difficulties do not translate to all women with Fibromyalgia.

With every baby I found the initial weeks painful, I experienced cracked and bleeding nipples by the end of the first week.

With my first, we found he was excessively windy and, by week two, we were going back and forward to doctors at the afterhours centre. At last, at week three, we were sent to the hospital, and there, they found that he had pyloric stenosis – a thickened sphincter that wouldn't let food out of the stomach to be digested, so it was forced back up and out of his mouth in projectile vomiting.

After several days in hospital and a small operation, we came home and found that he doubled the amount he was taking at each feed. My supply couldn't keep up, despite pumping three hourly the entire time he was in the hospital; my supply decreased in real numbers and relative numbers. I managed to keep him exclusively on breast milk until eight weeks. At this point, whenever it was time to express, I would cry, so I knew it was time to finish up. I was just tired and sore, and Noah was not a very settled baby and so cried the entire time I tried to express.

I was so relieved when parenting no longer needed to include my breasts. I am proud that I managed to give him such a good start in life. I also wish I had given up sooner, but the pressure on mothers to breastfeed is enormous, even my expressing rather than feeding directly was seen as failure. My doctor and my Plunket nurse were both supportive as they understood the Fibromyalgia and how hard I had tried.

With my second, I managed to persevere a little longer. My right breast got so sore and cracked from the second day cluster feeding that when I first tried to express, I expressed blood in the milk; it was a frightening sight. I persevered with the one side for another week before that became too sore (this guy was a rough feeder and liked to pull away with it clenched between his gums). I expressed four hourly during the day and once in the middle of the night (that was hard to leave baby sleeping after giving him a bottle and stay awake). My supply stayed static, no matter what I did to try to increase it, so, by week four, I was only just producing enough from both breasts for one feed. Luckily, I had a lot of frozen milk from the first weeks of expressing.

This time, I knew it didn't have to be all or nothing (this is an important message for all mamas; you can mix feed!); I had more knowledge and therefore more power. I also ignored any messages of my being deficient or not trying hard enough. I managed to add in a physical feed each evening after he had spent the previous few hours having more regular bottles in his nightly cluster feed, which meant I didn't have to worry about him not getting enough and he got some comfort from it at the end of a long day. It hurt, but swapping which breast I gave him each night helped me to cope. I worked with my midwife to reduce to a few feeds a day of my milk and add in formula for the shortfall. My plan was to give him whatever breast milk I could, for as long as I could.

As we know, plans do not always work out. Poor Wyatt developed reflux and vomited my milk and got very sore. Through long weeks of trial and error, we found that I could feed him directly (my measly 40 ml or so) followed immediately by a bottle of thickened formula, reducing the vomiting to spills and the gas pains greatly decreased. At seven weeks, I was still managing to mix feed, with the miniscule supply I produced.

Due to the very different positions in my health and a lot more knowledge and confidence, I believe it was slightly easier the second time around. However, by 12 weeks, my supply had completely dried up. I was really happy that I had been able to provide him with these vital nutrients for that long. I was also happy to not have to deal with expressing, feeding and bottles; it had begun to feel like my whole life revolved around his feeding. And at this time, my life turned to revolving around his sleep, or lack of!

My third was by far my most successful, although it was not an easy road either. In the second week we realised the severe pain I was feeling was due to thrush. A few weeks after that I got mastitis and needed antibiotics, which didn't help the thrush. We got through all of these things and were still going strong at nine months – with no pain.

My tips would mirror what most nursing people are told:

- Try to rest as much as you can
- Try to eat as well as you can
- Drink lots of water
- Make yourself as comfortable as possible when you feed
- If you feel pain beyond those initial tricky weeks, seek help and if you feel you are being fobbed off, get a second opinion. Thrush will stop even a non-fibro mother in her breastfeeding tracks.

Know that whatever you manage to give your baby is awesome and that you cannot fail. You will be a great parent whether you feed physically, by expressed breast milk or by formula. A fed baby and a happy parent are both minimum requirements. (Your wellbeing counts as much as baby's – and don't let anyone tell you otherwise!)

Fourth Trimester: The First Months

After the work of pregnancy, labour and the first few days, the most beautiful thing you can do for your baby and your body is to rest. In places like India and Asia, women have a "lie in"; for a month, they stay in bed and focus only on baby. A Fourth Trimester to ease you and baby into life.

First and foremost, we need to be more caring towards ourselves. Pregnancy is a difficult time for even the healthiest women. Labour is hard. Adjusting to a tiny needy baby is a real test of endurance. So taking that time and not considering it business as usual is really important. Particularly when you have a chronic illness for which pain and fatigue are already an issue. You're likely to flare up post birth. Sleep deprivation is no friend to pain or fatigue.

In order to give us a fair chance at succeeding in the endurance race that is the first year of having a new baby, let's consider the first few weeks as necessary resting/adjusting/healing time.

Some Useful Tips for the Post-Birth Period

Consider day and night as feasible sleeping times – try to arrange it so that you're not reliant on medicines that stop you getting to sleep without them. You may like to distinguish between night and day for baby: daytime feedings in the light, talking and singing, night-time feedings in dimmer light and more quiet.

- Sip on bone broth/soup broth for extra nutrients.
- Eat as best you can, despite potentially being too tired and sore to feel hungry. Consider smoothies with fruit and vegetables.
- Stay hydrated.
- Pelvic floor exercises!
- Let dad/partner/parent/friend take baby so you can rest and shower and eat and just be.
- Consider meditation for a nice booster (I love a guided meditation style called Yoga Nidra – 20 minutes is worth a few hours of sleep – and you can save varying lengths to your phone. Prayer is also meditative.)
- If you're breastfeeding, be wary of posture, hydration and fuel – it takes more energy than you may have.
- If you feel breastfeeding is a kick in the pants after your previous ordeals, as I did with Noah (far too painful and exhausting), don't feel guilty. You need to look after this baby and you for a long time yet, try to sense how much you can cope with before meltdown. Know that whatever you can give is beneficial. There are multiple options available to you.
- Switch between a comfortable chair/couch and your bed so your body doesn't get too sore from the same position.

- Jot down notes for your memory – I took many photos, videos and notes that I love looking back at.
- Store up some movies or TV series you might like to watch on some lazy days or when you're feeding.
- Have any supplements/medicines that you couldn't have while pregnant (and can have if breastfeeding) on hand, so that they're ready for you.
- Don't be too impatient to wean yourself off pain killers too fast. I forced myself off too soon with Noah thinking it was better to be less reliant on medicine, but I was only denying myself perfectly acceptable coping mechanisms.

How to get Through the First Six Weeks with a Baby, Fibromyalgia, Chronic Pain & Chronic Fatigue

It's "normal" to be really tired and sore after you have a baby, so, for the first time in my life, after my first baby, I experienced a few weeks of real support. It was an excruciating process to get my precious baby boy and the hard work hadn't finished yet!

After 37 weeks of increasingly sleepless, pain-filled weeks of pregnancy, I had no idea the worst was not yet over. A somewhat traumatic labour produced a beautiful baby boy who proceeded to ensure I didn't sleep for three nights. Stitches in a delicate place, profound exhaustion (that even several years with chronic fatigue cannot prepare you for), bruised and cracked nipples, a screaming baby that you don't yet know how to comfort and the traditional, almost lifelong neck and back pain abounded. But I survived.

Here are my recommendations for coping in the first six weeks:

I wouldn't have gotten through labour, let alone the first few weeks, without my husband; he helped me in the middle of the night, taking the 9.30pm – 12 shift most nights to enable me a jump start on the night with a few hours' sleep under my belt, and was generally a really great man. I know these tend to be in short supply – I have experienced the frogs before my prince – but I really could not have coped without him. Get a support person!

An important off-shoot of this: **try to give birth in a facility that enables your support person to stay the night with you.** It's a two-person job, and when you are dealing with the pain levels that hit you after labour, you need 24-hour support or you will crash on the third day, like I did; I spent the whole day crying. This is when the birthing centre relented and let my husband stay. There is a whole other marathon to go, and starting off so behind makes it much harder than it needs to be. With my second I refused to let my husband leave and it was good. By far the best decision I made was to go home as soon as possible after my third, without staying a night. That was wise.

Find the way that works for you when it comes to feeding this child you worked so hard to produce. For me with my first, that was expressing my milk and feeding him by bottle. There were several reasons breastfeeding physically didn't work for us as I wrote about earlier, but I only survived by being able to leave my husband or mum to feed baby and snatching precious snippets of sleep. Initially, my husband let me sleep for several hours in a row, which were vital in assisting my recovery. The consequence of this is that when I was alone with baby during the day, I had to fit in expressing every four hours, whether he was calm or not.

Have a really great extended support system. With my first, my mother took two weeks off work to be with me after my husband went back to work. After every baby, my mother-in-law cooked meals for us for the first few weeks and continued to make me a special semolina porridge mixture to assist with milk production. My husband's mum, dad, brother and sister were instrumental in allowing us to feel supported, but leaving us space to find our way. My brother Luke came to stay and help me out with the children often.

Sleep when you can. I love my bed. I spend far too little time there since I had children, but the typically spouted advice of "sleep when your baby sleeps" didn't work for me – my baby seemed to have a sixth sense for when I was trying to nap! But when my husband offered to do the late night feed, as soon as I expressed, I hit the sheets. When my mum popped over for an afternoon, I ran to my room.

Look after yourself. It's like the warning on the aeroplanes, put your own oxygen mask on before helping others – you are no good to that baby if you can't function.

Force yourself to eat; you need the energy. In the first week after my first was born, I was too exhausted to feel hungry, to contemplate what to eat, and I hardly wanted to perform the act of eating. But the longer I went, the more lethargic I felt and the less I was able to do. However, as I got into breastfeeding and eating again (extremely bland food such as marmite sandwiches got me going), I began to feel ravenous.

Have a shower or bath every day. Get dressed every day, even if it's yoga pants or just a clean pair of pyjama pants.

Take a walk as soon as you're able, start your pelvic floor exercises immediately – the blood flow assists healing and ensuring your muscles don't get too weak will help to avoid increased pain levels.

Conclusion

I followed all of these guidelines with my second and third babies and they were better experiences, despite both having reflux and struggling to sleep.

Necessary Baby Items for a Fibro Parent

There are a multitude of nursery items and almost as many articles about which ones are necessary. Here's my recommendations for a fibro mama, or really, any mama!

Below are some the items I found indispensable for a mama with fibromyalgia:

Bassinet

None of the options we used ended up being my favourite. For my second we used a Moses basket with a rocking base that we could move in and out of the bedroom so it was the best of the three. For my third we borrowed a rocking bassinet that I put beside my bed, the rocking ability was awesome, being unable to move the bassinet easily was not. My ideal would have been a bedside bassinet, especially one with a side that drops down so that you can easily move baby in and out from bed.

Changing Table

We weren't going to buy one. I had thought that I could get by without one. However, being given one has been a lifesaver. I have everything I need to change baby on the shelf and could lay them down at the right height for changing.

A Nursing Chair

My husband and I clashed about this one. He didn't think it was necessary. I believed with all my heart that it was. I ended up getting a second-hand one, and it was so useful. For nursing, expressing or just rocking when you're too tired to stand, it was worth it.

Pushchair

I recommend an easy to steer, lightweight pushchair with a small basket for carrying supplies. Getting it in and out of the car and folding it up needs to be easy, especially if you're sore.

Infant Capsule Seat with Folding Pushchair Frame

We didn't think we would use one because I thought it would be too heavy for me to lift. I was right: very quickly it became a real burden to carry. However, with the frame and the fact that baby could nap on the go, it turned out to be invaluable. The seat and frame meant that I could seamlessly move from car to shops to car to home easily.

A Front Pack

This was invaluable with my second and his reflux as I spent a lot of time carrying him upright as well as keeping my arms free for Noah. At about six months my little guys became too heavy for my shoulders to bear for too long, so this one does have a short-term life span.

A Bath Seat

This meant that I didn't have to hold their weight while they were in the bath and it was far easier to wash them.

Jolly Jumper

This was lovely for me when baby was super fussy and I was super tired. It gave me ten minutes of time out from holding them.

Portacot

We didn't get one until Noah was eight months old as we thought it was unnecessary once he outgrew the bassinet stage. We were wrong. It has been invaluable. Noah finally got the hang of proper napping at about eight months old (coinciding with our buying the portacot, but not because of it!), which means he needed to be able to sleep for 1-2 hours each morning and afternoon. The portacot meant that my boy could sleep at either grandparents' house, so we didn't have to squish a visit in between naps or push out naps.

One thing they can use to pull themselves up with

When Noah started to develop the ability to pull himself up, we got a table type toy where he could stand and play. This is a useful thing to let them stand without you holding them.

Baby (bumbo) Seat

This was something I wanted but didn't purchase until Noah was already sitting on his own. It would have been useful before this as he loved to sit and see so it could have bought me more non-holding time. For a long time, we used it strapped to a chair as his highchair. It is perfect for travel if you are driving to your destination.

Bouncinette/Electronic Rocker

This was one of those things that buys you some non-holding time that you so desperately need when they're clingy or your sore or you need to get stuff done.

Tips to Cope with a Fussy Baby When You're Sore

It's hard enough to be a parent with a fussy baby, let alone when you're in pain and beyond exhausted. Having a new baby is a soul-stretching time, you find the bottom of your energy reserves. They require a lot of love, time, energy and guesswork.

When your baby is fussy and you can't fix it (they're not hungry, windy, have a dirty nappy, and so on), and you're beside yourself.

Give these suggestions a try:

- **Sit on floor with them** – play with them, distract them with every toy you can think of. This will buy you some time and give your (possibly) aching shoulders a rest from carrying baby.
- **Take a gentle walk** – if they're soothed by the pushchair you can take a short walk. It might put them to sleep. Or at least give you some time off. You'll also get the benefits of fresh air.
- **Jolly jumper** – when they're big enough this can buy you another 10 minutes.
- **Rocking chair** – when you're too tired to jiggle and sway this is a lifesaver!

- **Swaddle and lie down** – when your reserves are at the end and you're too sore to try the rocking, swaying or singing anymore, swaddle baby tightly and lie down. Whether they're in their cot or with you in bed.

If they're not going to sleep or calm down and you need more rest, stay in bed for 15 minutes. You can't care for the baby if you're over your limit.

And please remember it will pass. They will grow up and the inexplicable crying will pass. You'll make it!

Coping with a Toddler: Fibromyalgia or Not!

Toddlers seem to have an abundance of energy that I could only dream of. If only they would lend me some – maybe it would be easier.

The big thing for me (on the days that I'm not working) is to get them active in the morning, when I'm most able and they're not so tired either. This way, the afternoon can be a more relaxed affair.

I am slowly learning that I'll never feel like I'm coping if I'm putting too much of my energy elsewhere (like work), so my balance needs to be kept in check.

Here's a few tips I've gleaned in dealing with two toddlers:

1. Accept help – my husband takes a turn in the morning when he's not at work. I never get back to sleep, but it's a break. If grandparents want to visit, give them the toddler and run away!

2. Enjoy them – this may be the sweetest age: Noah said things like, "Want some mama hug."

3. Play dough, stickers, colouring in to keep them occupied for 10 minutes.

4. Outside – even checking the mail and watering the garden can seem exciting.

5. Park – even if you need to drive there, the park is a great and free way to burn off toddler energy.

6. Routine – Noah is a routine boy and we have a loose but similar routine for each night; this helped when bedtime got foggy at the sleep regression. Wyatt is not so much a routine boy, but the framework keeps us on track.

7. Setting – first thing, before you get them up, set up some of their toys seductively. This may buy 10 minutes of independent play! I also swap toys around regularly.

8. Rest when the toddler (and baby) rests (if you're home with them) – on the days I'm home I will do Yoga Nidra meditation before anything else when the kids nap.

9. Library, zoo, beach, local attractions – there are options for all energy ranges. Noah loves animals, so we've been to the zoo a few times.

10. Read – when you're super exhausted and sore, lie or sit down (surrounded by cushions if need be) and read all of their books.

11. Movies – Noah wouldn't sit through anything longer than a minute at this age, but if this diversion works for your kids, then lie down immediately!

12. Play dates – another energetic creature can occupy yours! Mamas can chat. Win-win.

13. Pick your battles. Save your energy for the ones that count.

14. Consistency, set boundaries and always stick to them.

15. Don't forget yourself, keep experimenting and keep practicing your wellness techniques.

The last few are the result of a thread on my Facebook page, some amazing fibro mamas gave me some advice:

1. Educational games on a tablet – lie down and rest while they sit with you and play.

2. Have a bath together – get some toys or bath paints and let them play while you enjoy the warmth on your muscles.

3. Create a toddler-proof room that you can let them free and self-direct their play, sit back and enjoy their gorgeousness. (Do you do that? I've been known to stare at my boys and just grin.)

4. Don't always tidy up. The toys will be back out! Sometimes let the laundry and dishes be.

5. Take time out. Go for a coffee alone. Or a massage. Or a walk. Just go!

Mostly, I think having a toddler is a bit like a new-born in that you might need to just put your head down and push through. However, there are definitely more tools in the arsenal to keep them occupied once they clear babyhood.

Dear Significant Others to Fibro Parents

Congratulations!

This is going to be such a soul-stretching, exciting time in your life. Your relationship will be tested and strengthened. You'll learn more about yourself in these months than your whole life combined.

I have a request for you. Please, please, please be your partner's champion. Support them in their pregnancy. You'll never know the pain and energy drain that pregnancy is. But try to be compassionate.

Be their rock in the delivery. They will be in the worst pain imaginable. You need to be the safety in their storm. There will be decisions to make and there may be people you need to remove from the room. Do your homework, solidify your partner's wishes beforehand and try to help them stick to them (unless it's them who want to change!).

In the first few weeks at home with your precious, potentially persistently crying bundle, be your partner's superhero. They are recovering from delivery, learning to feed, and beyond exhausted and there will be a deluge of well-meaning advice.

Be the guard dog. Limit visitors. Avoid them in the first two weeks if you can. And limit their time while they're there. Watch your partner. If they seem tired or like they just want to deal with the baby without prying eyes, send them off.

Be their advocate. No matter how you choose to feed your baby, advocate for them. Support this. Yes, breast milk is best. But there are many options and it is a two-person relationship – parent and baby are equally important here.

If breastfeeding doesn't work or your partner hates it or your baby doesn't take to it – whatever reason, then you support the formula route too.

It is your job to protect them from the people that would give their two cents worth. Choose your people to listen to and help your partner say, "We're following the advice of... [GP, midwife, Plunket nurse, mother, etc.]."

Your attitude and your support will be vital for your new fibro parent. If they must fight you too, it will be the hardest time in the world for them. They won't enjoy it. They won't feel loved. They'll feel alone. There will be some fluctuating hormones. This is the time to support them and honour their feelings. If they cry, hold them. If they feel bombarded, fix it. If they feel happy, celebrate with them.

Of course, you're important too. I'm just offering the perspective of a new mama with Fibromyalgia. What I wished for myself and didn't always get.

Good luck!

The Best Ways You & Your Loved One Can Support You with Small Children & Fibromyalgia

Ordinarily, when your children are small, you expect a certain level of sleep deprivation and fatigue. When this is combined with moderate chronic insomnia, chronic pain and chronic fatigue, it's tough. In addition to good self-care habits, support from your loved one and good self-care habits will be invaluable.

For the first few weeks with Noah, Husband stayed up for the last few feeds so that I could get a jump start on sleep. Those precious four or so hours really made a difference. Unfortunately, the recognition of my insomnia, pain and fatigue seemed to level off after several months and life intervened – Husband is a shift worker and I had to work.

So I had to put some habits in place to protect myself.

I created a slow, gentle morning routine so we can transition into the day with less pain.

I began meditating most days for 20-30 minutes.

I have made hard choices; I said no to travelling to India while Noah was 1 year and 9 months old – travelling to India would be a big deal alone, but with a small child, it would be stupidity, especially if no one understands the impact of the pain, fatigue and sleeplessness. One gastro bug and I'd be wiped. I hate to think the impact of a severe gastro bug on a child so small.

I ask for the occasional morning off. I can't necessarily sleep in, but I can take a break from getting the children ready before I get to sit with my heat pack and coffee.

I'm very careful about the number of late nights we have, given that I'm exhausted by 9pm every night, children wake early and I can't nap. There isn't much wiggle room. The nights we do stay out late or have people over late, I am always more sore and tired the next day, and if I'm particularly sore, I sleep even worse.

I utilise my in-laws offer to have the children some days

Some things your loved one can do to support you include:

- Take turns getting up to small children/babies at night and early in the morning.
- Take turns cooking dinner.
- Not complain about the state of the house, notice what was done (and imagine how hard that was with three kids and chronic pain!).
- Remind you of your self-care necessities and give you space to enact them (a 30 minute lie down, a gentle walk, a hot bath etc.).
- Understand when you say you can't do something.
- Be open to modifications if you ask. For example, when considering travelling, support to put some mechanisms in place to

make it less difficult (otherwise, you'll be miserable and potentially worse for several months), things like ensuring a comfortable sleep environment, not sharing a room with loud toddlers, access to food that won't upset the tummy, not too many late nights and not going to the opposite side of the world for the first time with two very small children.

- Support you with the amount of hours you can work, balancing the illness and family responsibilities. Including encouragement to take the full year off after Baby (if possible).

- Notice how hard you try and thank you for all you do (it's not easy).

Of course, it's always good to try to focus on your relationship too. I try to tell Husband how thankful I am for him and how much I love him every day. We kiss every day. We try to have regular date times – even breakfast alone counts! I also do my best to accommodate the things he wants to do that go against my energy levels as often as possible.

The most important thing to remember is that the children aren't very small forever. Before we know it, they will be 3, then off to school, and then (eek) university! Once their demands on our night-time hour's decrease, things will be infinitely easier.

Resources

This is one of the only books written about pregnancy and Fibromyalgia. But here are some other resources that may be useful:

- Melissa vs Fibromyalgia blog (there is a large collection of articles I have written about pregnancy and parenting with Fibromyalgia)
- Pregnancy and Fibromyalgia Facebook Group (where we chat pregnancy, trying to conceive and nursing every day)
- Being Fibro Mom website (run by an awesome mama, Brandi Clevinger, with school age children)
- Fibro Parenting Facebook Group (run by the same amazing lady above)
- Mamas Facing Forward Facebook Group

Further Support

If you would like to work with a Fibromyalgia and Mindfulness Coach who has been through this (three times!) then please contact me to schedule a complimentary chat to discuss where you are at, what your goals are and how coaching might help you.

Summary of November 2017 Research Survey

During November 2017, I sent a survey via Google Forms with nine questions. I sought responses via a post on my blog and a link on several social media forums. 21 people responded.

Did you find pregnancy made your symptoms worse or better?

Better – 52.4%   *Worse – 47.6%*

Did you experience a severe flare up after the birth of your baby?

Yes – 68.4%   *No – 31.6%*

Did you manage to nurse?

No – 15.8%   *For 12 months – 21.1%*

For six months – 21.1%   *For more – 36.8%*

Exclusive expressing – 5.2%

Summary of February 2018 Research Survey

During February 2018, I sent a survey via Google Forms with nine questions. I sought responses via a post on my blog and a link on several social media forums I participate in. And twenty people responded.

Short Answer Questions:

Do you have Fibromyalgia?

    Yes – 100%   No – 0%

Did you find that your pain was worse during pregnancy?

    Yes – 70%   No – 30%

What main medicine did you take during pregnancy?

    None – 35%   Gabapentin – 10%

    Antidepressant – 5%   Anti-nausea meds – 5%

    Acetaminophen – 25%

    Medicine not directly related to Fibromyalgia – 20%

What was your favourite pain relief mechanism during pregnancy?

1. Warm baths/showers and rest were the top choices
2. Chiropractic care
3. Epsom salts
4. Massage
5. Ice pack
6. Essential oils

Paragraph Questions:

Kristen's advice

How did you manage your pain/fatigue during pregnancy?

The pain was way better. I just took naps and hot baths.

How did you manage in those early weeks with baby?

I used a lot of ibuprofen, hot baths, and massage. I'm 5 months [at the time] postpartum and it's really bad now. Only thing that helps temporarily is massage and hot baths.

Do you have any advice for other fibro parents about parenting with Fibromyalgia?

I have to rest a lot. I made sure I was with someone that would truly help out with the kids. He takes over at night with the baby so I can sleep. Sleep is essential!

Marlene's advice

How did you manage your pain/fatigue during pregnancy?

I was fortunate that my job had flexible hours, so I napped whenever I could. I limited my caffeine, didn't take medication except Tylenol, took long baths and began prepping way ahead of time, also cut myself a break whenever possible. Takeout food!

How did you manage in those early weeks with baby?

Rest! Take Tylenol if you need it. Take baths but not too hot...doctor said that hot wasn't good for the baby. Begin prepping asap, also cut yourself a break whenever possible. Order good Takeout food!

Do you have any advice for other fibro parents about parenting with Fibromyalgia?

It's really tough to do it all, if you can get family help that doesn't stress you out, do it. If you don't have that option get a mother's helper when the baby is a little older. Mainly rest when the baby rests, leave the dishes, order takeout, place your grocery order online and pick up at store or pay for delivery that is your number 1 time and body saver! Use Amazon to save yourself from running around and running yourself down. Join a new baby group.... hospitals sometimes have these.

Victoria's advice

How did you manage your pain/fatigue during pregnancy?

Rest, a lot

How did you manage in those early weeks with baby?

I ended up feeling great after giving birth. Relaxed or slept anytime the baby was asleep.

Do you have any advice for other fibro parents about parenting with Fibromyalgia?

Know your limitations. Talk to your kids early. Find ways to play that don't involve a ton of movement. Read to them. One of my daughter's favorite activities is lying next to me as I read to her.

A Fibro Parent's advice

How did you manage your pain/fatigue during pregnancy?

Napping as much as possible, prenatal yoga, prenatal massage. Honestly though my pain hasn't been that low in years

How did you manage in those early weeks with baby?

Fresh ginger and lemon in hot water, crackers, prenatal yoga, fizzy decaf drinks, French bread, clementines, family support (had a scary start)

Do you have any advice for other fibro parents about parenting with Fibromyalgia?

Sleep when you can. Never feel bad about napping when the baby/toddler/big kid is napping. Have your partner bring the baby to you to nurse. I leave my heating pad on my chair 24/7. I went down to 32 hours a week of work which still gives me full time benefits.

Casey's advice

How did you manage your pain/fatigue during pregnancy?

Rest, warm baths

How did you manage in those early weeks with baby?

Dad helped a lot.

A Fibro Parent's advice

How did you manage your pain/fatigue during pregnancy?

Heat, ice, neurontin

How did you manage in those early weeks with baby?

My fibromyalgia was still in very early stages then, and after my daughter was born it was a lot better.

Robbyn's advice

How did you manage your pain/fatigue during pregnancy?

I took a lot of hot showers, used heating pads, stretched and walked, a lot.

How did you manage in those early weeks with baby?

A lot of rest, snuggling baby, getting help from Daddy to do housework because I really couldn't get much of any of that done.

Do you have any advice for other fibro parents about parenting with Fibromyalgia?

Rest when you can. Have lazy days, where you snuggle and watch movies with the kids. We have a lot of lazy days on the weekends where we have popcorn and movie parties in my bed because everything just hurts too much to do much else.

Krista's advice

How did you manage your pain/fatigue during pregnancy?

I took a lot of naps!! The only thing I could do for the pain was Tylenol and I took that very sparingly.

How did you manage in those early weeks with baby?

I slept when the baby slept. We didn't go places, we stayed home and just got acclimated to each other.

Do you have any advice for other fibro parents about parenting with Fibromyalgia?

Just try your best. It might not be easy at times but it will all be worth it. If you have a bad day, rest. And then on good days, do something special with your kids like going to the park. Grant yourself grace!

Danielle's advice

How did you manage your pain/fatigue during pregnancy?

I slept and rested more than when I wasn't pregnant. I was undiagnosed at the time of my pregnancies, but knew I had to rest way more to ensure that I was healthy enough to carry my babies to term. I followed my body's signs and rested if I needed to.

How did you manage in those early weeks with baby?

Focused more on resting when I could. This included letting my husband and both sets of grandparents help with care and bottle feeding so I could rest and/or sleep when I needed to.

Do you have any advice for other fibro parents about parenting with Fibromyalgia?

If you need to rest, don't feel guilty about it. Plan when you will be using your energy. If you know you are going to do something with your kids, then plan to rest the day after. Don't be afraid to use medication if you need it. I wouldn't be able to be present for my kids or be as successful in my job without it.

A Fibro Parent's advice

How did you manage your pain/fatigue during pregnancy?

I slept as much as possible and did anything that was comforting. I tried to take a lot of baths and hot showers, eat small snacks to not get sick. I noticed my IBS symptoms were much worse.

How did you manage in those early weeks with baby?

As hard as it is, let the housework go. Sleep when you can and for as long as you can. Try to keep self-care at the front of your mind. Remembering to eat, shower, and do small things you enjoy (a special treat, seeing a friend, going to a movie). Also seek immediate help if you feel you have PPD.

Do you have any advice for other fibro parents about parenting with Fibromyalgia?

When you do feel well try to do things with your children. Simple things, bake cookies, watch a movie, read a book. But to also plan ahead for bad days. When you feel well set up busy boxes or activities children can get to themselves or with minimal set up to be ready for flare up days.

Sara's advice

How did you manage your pain/fatigue during pregnancy?

Healthy eating rest and stretching

How did you manage in those early weeks with baby?

Baby carrier, boppy, rest, lots of water, chiropractor

Do you have any advice for other fibro parents about parenting with Fibromyalgia?

Learn your limits, get sleep. Self-care is so important.

Nicola's advice

How did you manage your pain/fatigue during pregnancy?

The most important factor is to put yourself first, you must rest when you need to and live within your physical limits. Never go beyond what you're physically capable of as that makes everything worse

How did you manage in those early weeks with baby?

Drop all the expectations that you need to be 'super' you and baby come first. Put yours and babies needs first, there were many times I didn't feel well enough to go out of the house and I used to feel so guilty but now I look back I realise it never harmed my child but at the time I would compare myself to other mothers who were out and about socialising, working or at baby groups etc

Do you have any advice for other fibro parents about parenting with Fibromyalgia?

As long as kids are loved and cared for by you there's no major detriment to having a slightly differing lifestyle. Sometimes I'd be too ill to take them out to parks etc and I'd feel so guilty but with hindsight they've grown to be happy well-adjusted etc. And it's ok now and again to feed them a meal that isn't cooked from scratch if you are feeling ill, drop any guilt and be kinder to yourself

Teana's advice

How did you manage your pain/fatigue during pregnancy?

I spent all my time in bed. I had two toddlers and was pregnant with the third child. My husband was in the military and I was basically on my own. I was really worried my other two kids would be damaged long term from the time we had to be confined to one room so that I could manage them and take care of them. I made a game of cleaning, had them race and timed them. We watched a lot of cartoons and read a lot of books. I learned that it was about time you spend with them rather than the actual activity you do.

How did you manage in those early weeks with baby?

It was a nightmare honestly, I would fall asleep during feedings and spill precious breast milk all over myself, my kid, and my bed. So I had to give up breast feeding early with her. I asked for a lot of help, any family member that could come and entertain the other two, my husband when he was home did all the work with the kids so I could 'catch up' on my rest. I use quotations there because even moms without this disease never catch up on rest. If you don't have a lot of help, making sure to take as much time as you need to rest and then only doing what absolutely had to be done on the days you feel better was the key for me.

Do you have any advice for other fibro parents about parenting with Fibromyalgia?

It gets both easier and harder as they grow up. My oldest are both teens now and them along with the 'baby' help me tremendously. They do most of the light housework and even some heavy stuff when my husband is home and able to help. My daughters and I use weird times, like them helping me dress and wash my hair or they offer massages for my back and feet, to connect and talk about their days and what's going on with them. Kids care if you're there for them, not how much you can do. They are smart and they know if you are hurt. My oldest daughter comforted me when I had to ask her to help me wash my hair, she said, "Momma, you did all this for me when I couldn't do it, why wouldn't I do it for you?"

A Fibro Parent's advice

How did you manage your pain/fatigue during pregnancy?

Paracetamol and a microwave pillow, and lots of backrubs. To be honest I didn't have much success managing my pain, I was in pain for a lot of the time, my mobility was very limited and it was pretty horrible. This has played a big part in my decision not to have any more children.

How did you manage in those early weeks with baby?

The pain improved a good deal once I gave birth. Thinking back, I wish I had tried to outsource more of the work at home (used a laundry service/hired a cleaner) but I just didn't think of it. I think that would have helped with my overwhelming stress.

Do you have any advice for other fibro parents about parenting with Fibromyalgia?

Get diagnosed/medicated before you start trying for a family. I really wish I had done that.

Hannah's advice

How did you manage your pain/fatigue during pregnancy?

Chiropractor, massage, acupuncture, and sleep/rest

How did you manage in those early weeks with baby?

Lots of help from family and husband, found breastfeeding very tiring and strain on neck and back so had to use support aids or lay in bed to feed. Naps when baby napped were crucial. Treated myself to dark chocolate or some snack as often as possible while feeding baby so I was doing self-care. Gentle walks and yoga were good too.

Do you have any advice for other fibro parents about parenting with Fibromyalgia?

You can't pour from an empty cup, but with fibromyalgia you almost always feel empty, but you can do this. Remember self-care is taking care of your baby in long run and that you know what works and is right for you so please take all advice on board but don't think it's the law and has to be used. Also mother groups it's okay to not like them I hated them or didn't find the right mums doesn't mean you're alone though we fibromyalgia are probably all just online so talk to us! I also think this time round I'm writing a list of helpful jobs people can do for me with as I found it difficult asking for help and people may not know what to offer and you might be so tired in pain you can't properly communicate. So I'm hoping just having a help task list might be a good compromise. It also something my husband a toddler can learn to look at together on weekends maybe.

Elizabeth's advice

How did you manage your pain/fatigue during pregnancy?

I survived 3 pregnancies through pure determination, lots of essential oils, rest and help from friends and family. Finding a good doctor that understands that a chronic pain body's endorphins do not actually help with the pain is paramount. (This can be frustrating and difficult). Make sure you don't give into your cravings because often they will make your fibro flare.

How did you manage in those early weeks with baby?

Casseroles and family. Accept all the help that is offered and if you need more, ask! Most people don't want to step on toes but are more than happy to help, especially if there's a new baby. :) It's ok if your house isn't spick and span. If the laundry is washed, that can be good enough. Use paper plates to cut down on dishes. Be nice to yourself!! Cut yourself extra slack.

Do you have any advice for other fibro parents about parenting with Fibromyalgia?

Teach your children to be super helpers!

A Fibro Parent's advice

How did you manage your pain/fatigue during pregnancy?

Heat pads and taking it easy. I actually was better during the beginning of my pregnancy. I think all the extra estragon helped me feel better. I did have a lot of pain towards the end, but probably everyone does because of all the weight. My hubby noticed me happier and feeling better though, during most of it. I still thought I had pain though, but he said I complained less and definitely seemed in a better disposition. It was after the pregnancy that's when I had lots of pain from the birth, stress of being a new mom, and not being about to lift my child because of the pain.

How did you manage in those early weeks with baby?

Tried to eat right and listen to my body. I passed out from not enough protein in the beginning.

Do you have any advice for other fibro parents about parenting with Fibromyalgia?

Listen to your body and don't feel guilty about taking a rest. You need to be your best for them and not stress out your body.

Caroline's advice

How did you manage your pain/fatigue during pregnancy?

Showers, massage, physical therapy, rest

How did you manage in those early weeks with baby?

Lots of help, showers

Do you have any advice for other fibro parents about parenting with Fibromyalgia?

Pay attention to the weather as it greatly affects fibro. Watch your diet, plan your days according to the weather, how much sleep you got, and what you eat. Nap at least once a day with your little ones.

Acknowledgements

Thank you to those few people I have met who have truly attempted to understand this beast I fight.

To the generous fibro fighters who share your advice in the amazing Facebook groups I am in and the wonderful women in my Pregnancy and Fibromyalgia group. You all inspire me.

Thank you to Luke for your friendship, for never saying no to helping me, whether it's with the children or making an image for the blog. And thanks for designing my book cover and making my book pretty.

Thank you to Husband, Noah, Wyatt and Nathaniel – my reason for living and fighting. I know it hasn't been easy on you, Husband, but I thank you for helping me to live the best life I can, despite the Fibromyalgia.

And thank you to my Lord Jesus Christ, without whom my footprints along the beach would have ceased long ago. Thank you for instilling this sense of mission in me that my work might help others.

About the Author

Melissa Reynolds has fought Fibromyalgia since she was 14 years old. Only, she didn't receive a name for her invisible opponent until she was in her 20s. Unfortunately, the name of the illness did not come with help.

After declaring war, she went from miserable and barely coping with life to thriving in seven years. Using a combination of research and personal trial and error, she has managed to bring her pain and fatigue levels down and minimise the effects of the debilitating brain fog. She shares her learning through coaching, in her books *Melissa vs Fibromyalgia: My Journey Fighting Chronic Pain, Chronic Fatigue and Insomnia, Fibromyalgia Framework Workbook* and *Pregnancy and Fibromyalgia*, and her Facebook groups Fibro Mama Pregnancy and Fibromyalgia and Melissa (you) vs Fibromyalgia.

Melissa lives in Auckland, New Zealand, with her family.

Before You Go

I hope this book has helped you. If you want to connect with me, you can find me:

- My blog: melissavsfibromyalgia.com (check out the *Resources* page with free resources and my Pregnancy Diaries and Resources page has all of my pregnancy-specific resources);
- Facebook group: Fibro Mama Pregnancy and Fibromyalgia;
- Email me to request your complimentary session to discuss where you are at, your goals and if coaching would help you melissa[at]melissavsfibromyalgia.com

And could I ask you a favour? Would you please post a review on the website where you purchased it and/or Goodreads? That way, we can make a start on filling the void that is information on pregnancy and Fibromyalgia.

References

Fibromyalgia and Pregnancy: The Literature

Jacob Teitelbaum, MD. (2013). *Pregnancy in Chronic Fatigue Syndrome and Fibromyalgia*. The Environmental Illness Resource. Retrieved from http://www.ei-resource.org/expert-columns/dr-jacob-teitelbaums-column/pregancy-in-chronic-fatigue-syndrome-and-fibromyalgia/

Kevin P. White (writer), & Kenneth R. Hirsch, MD (medically reviewed). (2014). *Fibromyalgia and Pregnancy: Expert Q&A*. Healthline. Retrieved from https://www.healthline.com/health/fibromyalgia-and-pregnancy-expert-qa

WebMD. (2016). *Fibromyalgia and Pregnancy*. WebMD. Retrieved from https://www.webmd.com/fibromyalgia/guide/fibromyalgia-and-pregnancy

National Fibromyalgia & Chronic Pain Association. (2014). *Tips for Pregnancy with Fibromyalgia*. National Fibromyalgia & Chronic Pain Association (NFMCPA). Retrieved from https://www.fmcpaware.org/tips-for-pregnancy-with-fibromyalgia.html

Malaika Babb, PharmD, Gideon Koren, MD, FRCPC, FACMT, & Adrienne Einarson, RN. (2010). *Treating Pain During Pregnancy*.

NCBI. Retrieved from
https://www.ncbi.nlm.nih.gov/pmc/articles/PMC2809170/

Monika Østensen, Anne Rugelsjoen, & Sigrid Horven Wigers. (1997). *The Effect of Reproductive Events and Alterations of Sex Hormone Levels on the Symptoms of Fibromyalgia*. Scandinavian Journal of Rheumatology, volume 26, issue 5. Retrieved from http://www.tandfonline.com/doi/abs/10.3109/03009749709065698 ?src=recsys

UK Teratology Information Service (UKTIS). (2014). *Amitriptyline* (Version 2). BUMPS (Best Use of Medicines in Pregnancy). Retrieved from http://www.medicinesinpregnancy.org/Medicine--pregnancy/Amitriptyline/

Fertility & Fibromyalgia: Not an Area of Concern, According to Research

Dr. Ananya Mandal, MD. (2013). *Fibromyalgia and Fertility/Pregnancy*. News Medical. Retrieved from https://www.news-medical.net/health/Fibromyalgia-and-Fertility-Pregnancy.aspx

Jacob Teitelbaum, MD. (2017). *Treating Infertility in Fibromyalgia – An Information Sheet for Couples*. ProHealth. Retrieved from http://www.prohealth.com/library/showarticle.cfm?libid=30232

Tiffany Vance-Huffman. (2017). *Fibromyalgia and Fertility.* Fibromyalgia Treating. Retrieved from http://www.fibromyalgiatreating.com/fibromyalgia-and-fertility/

Lots of Natural Pain Relief Suggestions

Christina Anthis. (2015). *Using Essential Oils Safely for Pregnant & Nursing Mamas.* The Hippy Homemaker. Retrieved from http://www.thehippyhomemaker.com/using-essential-oils-safely-for-pregnant-nursing-mamas/

Pain Management in Pregnancy with Fibromyalgia

Dr Abdul Lalkhen & Dr Kate Grady. (2008). *Non-Obstetric Pain in Pregnancy.* Retrieved from https://www.ncbi.nlm.nih.gov/pmc/articles/PMC4589928/

Drugs.com. (n.d.). *FDA Pregnancy Risk Information: An Updated.* Drugs.com. Retrieved from https://www.drugs.com/pregnancy-categories.html

Katarina Zulak. (2018). Pain, Pregnancy & Prescriptions: Why You Should Treat Your Pain And How To Manage Safely (While Trying To Conceive & Pregnant). Retrieved from https://skillfullywell.com/2018/04/19/pain-pregnancy-prescriptions-why-you-should-treat-your-pain-and-how-to-manage-safely-while-trying-to-conceive-pregnant/

LDN Science. (2016). *Interview with Phil Boyle*. Retrieved from https://www.ldnscience.org/resources/interviews/interview-phil-boyle

Malaika Babb, PharmD, Gideon, MD, FRCPC, FACMT, & Adrienne Einarson, RN. (2010). *Treating Pain During Pregnancy*. Can Fam Physcian, 56(1): 25, 27. Retrieved from https://www.ncbi.nlm.nih.gov/pmc/articles/PMC2809170/

Michael McCullough. (2011). *Analgesics and Pain Relief in Pregnancy and Breastfeeding*. Retrieved from https://www.nps.org.au/australian-prescriber/articles/analgesics-and-pain-relief-in-pregnancy-and-breastfeeding

Dr Nilesh Nolkha. (2018). Rheumatoid, psoriatic arthritis & pregnancy : All queries answered. Retrieved from https://www.arthritisrheumindia.com/rheumatoid-psoriatic-arthritis-pregnancy/

Dr Phil Boyle. (n.d.). *Low Dose Naltrexone In Pregnancy*. Retrieved from http://ldn2016.com/sites/default/files/Dr-Phil-Boyle.pdf

Pregnancy with Fibromyalgia: Tools for Managing Early Pregnancy Symptoms

Amy Maher. (2015). *Pregnancy Relaxation – Guided Meditation for Pregnancy Women*. YouTube. Retrieved from https://www.youtube.com/watch?v=954oDA7PTNk

Melissa Reynolds. (2016). *Giant Meditation Post*. Melissa vs Fibromyalgia (website). Retrieved from https://melissavsfibromyalgia.com/2016/03/19/giant-meditation-post/

Sarah Beth Yoga. (2016). *Top Three Yoga Poses for Pregnancy*. YouTube. Retrieved from https://www.youtube.com/watch?v=5XKaDOYUpiw

Erica Ziel. (2016). *5 Exercises to Help Get Rid of Back Pain During Pregnancy*. Knocked-Up Fitness. Retrieved from http://knocked-upfitness.com/5-exercises-to-help-get-rid-of-back-pain-during-pregnancy/

Nursing with Fibromyalgia

WebMD. (2014). Fibromyalgia Health Centre. WebMD. Retrieved from https://www.webmd.com/fibromyalgia/default.htm

Fibromyalgia Symptoms. (2017). *Breastfeeding with Fibromyalgia – Yes, It's Possible*. Retrieved from https://www.fibromyalgia-symptoms.org/nursing-and-fibromyalgia.html

Pregnancy with Fibromyalgia: Tools for Managing Early Pregnancy Symptoms

Amy Maher. (2015). *Pregnancy Relaxation – Guided Meditation for Pregnancy Women.* YouTube. Retrieved from https://www.youtube.com/watch?v=954oDA7PTNk

Made in the USA
Monee, IL
05 August 2020